Low Carb Recipes

For

One Person

Simple & delicious low carb recipes for one person

These one-dish recipes are super easy to prepare and even easier to clean up. Made with a diabetic menu in mind.

Table Of Contents

Table Of Contents
Terms Of Use Agreement
   Disclaimer
Delicious Wrapped Chicken
Pork & Cabbage Soup
Cauliflower Baked Twice
Simple Chicken For One
Light French Toast
Simple Scrambled Eggs
Carrot Pumpkin Bars
Spicy Chicken Soup
Joetta's Chile Lime Chicken Taco Salad
Low Carb Chili
Easy Beef Brisket
Beef Salad with Edamame
Low Carb Lobster Salad
Chinese Tuna Kebabs
Asparagus & Leek Soup
Asparagus & Tarragon Soup
Sausage Pizza With Bell Peppers and Onions
Low Carb Yorkshire Pudding

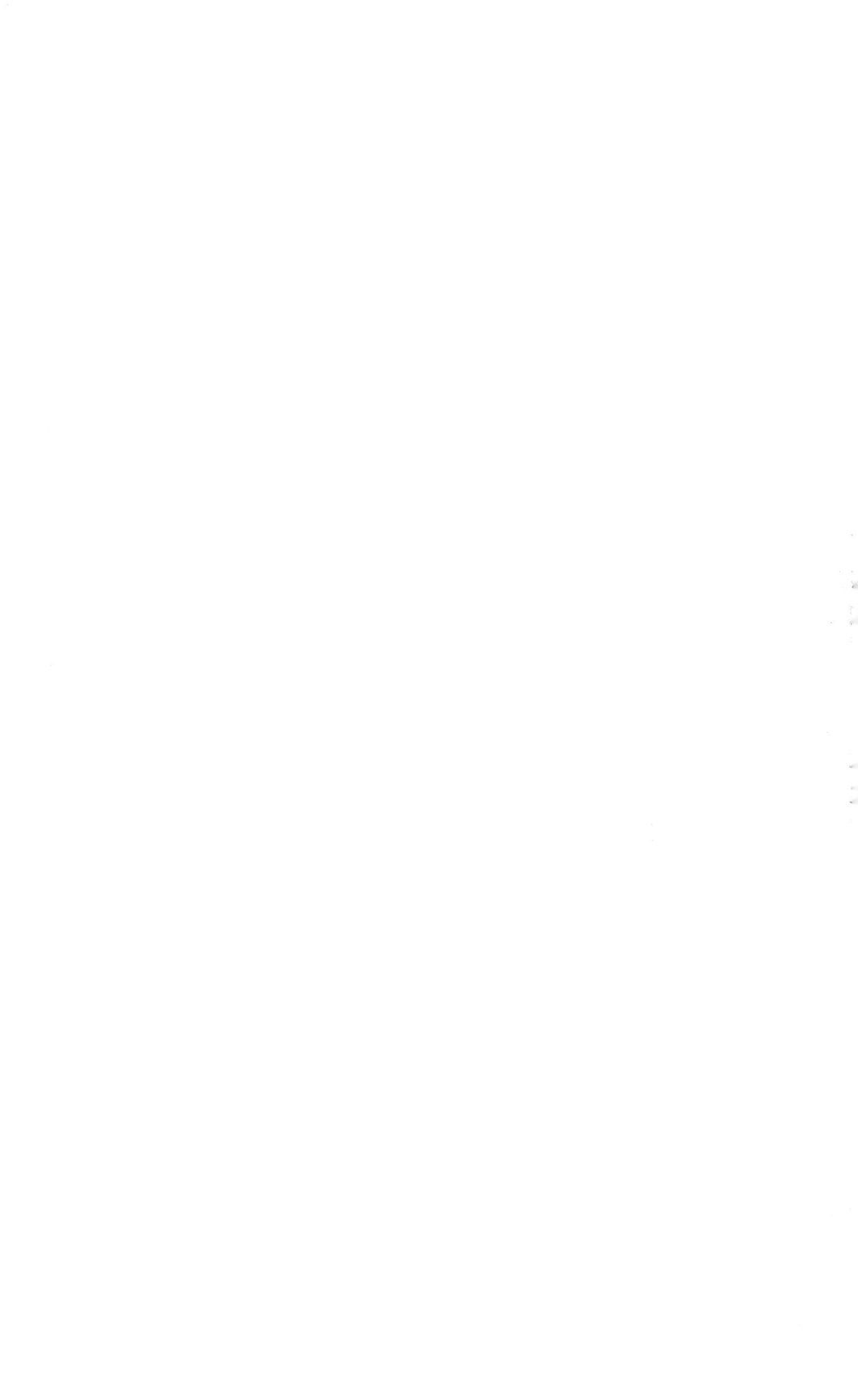

Terms Of Use Agreement

Copyright 2015
All Rights Reserved

The author hereby asserts his/her right to be identified as the author of this work in accordance with sections 77 to 78 of the copyright, design and patents act 1988 as well as all other applicable international, federal, state and local laws.

Without limiting the rights under copyright reserved above, no part of this book may be reproduced, stored in or introduced into retrieval system, or transmitted, in any form or by any electronic or mechanical means, without the prior written permission of the copyright owner of this book, except by a reviewer who may quote brief passages.

There are no resale rights included. Anyone re - selling, or using this material in any way other than what is outlined within this book will be prosecuted to the full extend of the law.

Every effort had been made to fulfill requirements with regard to reproducing copyrighted material. The author and the publisher will be glad to certify any omissions at the earliest opportunity.

Disclaimer

The author and the publisher have used their best efforts in preparing this book. The author and the publisher make no representation or warranties with respect to the accuracy, fitness, applicability, or completeness of the contents of this work and specifically disclaim all warranties, including without limitation warranties of fitness for a particular purpose. This work is sold with the understanding that author and the publisher is not engaged in rendering legal, or any other professional services.

The information contained in this book is strictly for educational purposes. Therefore, if you wish to apply ideas contained within this book, you are taking full responsibility for your actions. The author and the publisher disclaim any warranties (express or implied), merchantability, or fitness for any particular purpose.

The Author and The publisher shall in no event be held responsible / liable to any party for any indirect, direct, special, punitive, incidental, or other consequential damages arising directly or indirectly from any use of this material, which is provided 'as is', and without warranties.

The author and the publisher do not warrant the performance, applicability, or effectiveness of any websites and other medias listed or linked to in this publication. All links are for informative purposes only and are not warranted for contents, accuracy, or any other implied or explicit purpose.

Delicious Wrapped Chicken

Ingredients

- 4 oz. green beans
- 2 tsp. olive oil
- Coarse salt and ground pepper
- 1 boneless, skinless chicken breast half
- 3 thin slices prosciutto
- 1 wedge lemon

Directions

- Heat broiler or toaster oven. On rimmed baking sheet, toss green beans with 1 teaspoon oil.
- Season with salt and pepper, and push to one side of pan.
- Season chicken with salt and pepper; wrap with prosciutto.
- Place chicken, seam side down, on other side of pan; rub with remaining teaspoon oil.
- Broil until chicken is opaque throughout, 15 to 20 minutes.
- Serve with a lemon wedge.

- Enjoy!

Pork & Cabbage Soup

Ingredients

- 1/2 head Cabbage
- 1 lb lean pork tenderloin, cooked and shredded
- 1 can diced tomatoes
- Salt to taste
- Southwest seasoning
- 2 cups chicken stock
- 2 cups water

Directions

- Cook pork in crock pot, oven, or bbq smoker, seasoned with southwest seasoning.
- Chop 1/2 head cabbage
- Add 2 cups of chicken stock to medium saucepan bring to boil, add chopped cabbage and southwest seasoning, cook for 10 minutes, add pork and canned tomatoes, cook until cabbage is tender
- Enjoy!

Cauliflower Baked Twice

Ingredients

- 1 large head cauliflower
- 4 oz. low fat cream cheese
- 1 T butter
- 1/2 cup fat free sour cream
- 1/4 cup minced green onions
- 1/4 cup freshly grated Parmesan cheese
- 5 slices bacon, cooked very crisp and crumbled
- 1 cup reduced fat sharp cheddar cheese

Directions

- Preheat oven to 350 F. Cut out stem and core from cauliflower, and cut into small pieces. Cook in large pot of boiling water until cauliflower is tender, but not overly soft.
- Drain well and mash with potato masher, leaving some chunks. Mix in cream cheese, butter , sour cream, green onion, Parmesan, and 3/4 of the bacon.

- Spread evenly in an 8 X 8 inch glass casserole dish. Sprinkle with cheddar cheese and reserved bacon.
- Bake 30-35 minutes, or until hot and bubbly.
- Enjoy!

Simple Chicken For One

Ingredients

- 1 skinless chicken breast
- cooking spray
- salt
- pepper, freshly ground
- 1 teaspoon paprika

Directions

- Preheat oven to 400 F .
- Sprinkle salt and pepper over both sides of chicken.
- Spray chicken all over with cooking spray.
- Sprinkle with paprika.
- Place chicken bone side down on roaster rack.
- Roast for approximately 45 minutes or until juices run clear.
- Enjoy!

Light French Toast

Ingredients

- 2 slices whole wheat bread
- 1/4 cup milk (nonfat)
- 1/2 cup egg beaters
- tsp cinnamon
- tsp vanilla extract
- tsp splenda

Directions

- Mix together all ingredients in a bowl (except bread)
- Dip each slice of bread on each side into mixture.
- Coat pan with nonstick spray & turn stove on med/low heat.
- Place in pan for approximately 3-4 mins on each side.
- Serve and enjoy!

Simple Scrambled Eggs

Ingredients

- 2 large eggs
- 2 tablespoons of cold tap water
- 1 tablespoons whipped butter
- salt
- pepper

Directions

- In a mixing bowl crack 2 large eggs into the bowl
- Add 2 tablespoons of cold tap water.
- Beat together,
- Place 1 tablespoons of whipped butter into non stick pan.
- Cook over medium heat and stir constantly.
- Season and enjoy!

Carrot Pumpkin Bars

Ingredients

- Filling:
- 2 cups flour
- 1 1/4 teaspoon pumpkin pie spice
- 2 teaspoon baking powder
- 1 teaspoon baking soda
- 1 cup sugar
- 1/3 cup light butter/margarine, softened
- 1/2 cup brown sugar
- 2 eggs
- 2 large egg whites
- 1 can (15 oz.) pumpkin pie filling
- 1 cup carrot, finely shredded
-
- Cream cheese topping:
- 4 oz light cream cheese, softened
- 1/4 cup sugar
- 1 tablespoon skim milk

Directions

- Pre-heat oven to 350.

- Grease jelly roll pan.
- Prepare Filling:
- In small bowl: combine flour, pumpkin spice, baking powder & baking soda.
- In larger bowl: Beat sugar, butter and brown sugar until crumbly. Add eggs, egg whites, pumpkin pie mix and carrots. Beat until well blended. Add flour mixture and mix until well blended. Spread onto greased pan.
- Prepare Cream Cheese topping:
- Mix together cream cheese, sugar and milk until thoroughly blended.
- Drop teaspoon-fulls of topping over pumpkin batter and swirl mixture with a butter knife.
- Bake for 25-30 minutes.
- Cool in pan completely on wire rack before cutting into squares.
- Enjoy!

Spicy Chicken Soup

Ingredients

- 3 chicken breasts
- 2 cans of chicken broth
- 1 can black beans
- 1 can diced tomatoes
- 1/2 onion-chopped
- 1 jalapeno-chopped
- 1 tbsp minced garlic

Directions

- Makes 8 severing of one cup. For a heartier meal serves 4 servings of 2 cups.
- Prepare chicken to liking (taco seasoning) in pan
- Set chicken aside to cool and shred
- In large pot spray bottom lightly with PAM and cook chopped onions, jalapenos, and garlic
- Add chicken, 2 cans broth, 1/2 can water, tomatoes, and beans
- Add seasoning to taste (oregano, garlic powder, pepper, chili powder-1 tsp)
- Stir, boil and serve

- Enjoy!

Joetta's Chile Lime Chicken Taco Salad

Ingredients

- 3 oz. Boneless, skinless chicken breast
- 1 oz. Lime juice
- 1 Tbsp. Stubb's Chile Lime seasoning
- 1/2 tsp. ground cumin
- Dash of Adobo seasoning
- 1 1/2 cup Romaine lettuce
- 1/2 cup Spinach
- 1/3 cup Canned black beans (drained, rinsed)
- 3 tbsp salsa
- 2 tbsp fat free sour cream
- 1/4 avocado (sliced)
- 1 oz. Tostitos light tortilla chips

Directions

- Cut up chicken into chunks and brown in a pan using cooking spray. Add lime juice and spices and continue cooking chicken until done.

- Toss romaine and spinach in a big bowl. Add chicken chunks, black beans, salsa, sour cream, and avocado cut into slices. Sprinkle with crushed tortilla chips.
- Enjoy!

Low Carb Chili

Ingredients

- 1/8 medium (2-1/2" dia) Onion
- 8 oz boneless Steak
- 1/3 tbsp Chili Powder
- 1/16 tsp Black Pepper
- 1/4 tsp Salt
- 1 1/2 ozs Red Tomatoes (with Green Chilies, Canned)
- 1/4 tsp Garlic
- 2/3 fl oz Red Table Wine
- 1/3 tbsp Extra Virgin Olive Oil

Directions

- Cooking evaporates alcohol, which is why this recipe is suitable for Induction despite the red wine.
- But feel free to use chicken broth instead.
- Jarred roasted garlic cloves can be found in the produce section of most supermarkets.
- Heat oven to 325°F.

- Toss beef with salt and pepper.
- Heat 1 1/2 teaspoons oil in a Dutch oven over high heat.
- Add one-third of the beef and brown on all sides, about 5 minutes.
- Transfer to a bowl and repeat two more times with beef and oil.
- Add the last 1 1/2 teaspoons oil to Dutch oven and cook onion until lightly browned.
- Stir in chili powder, tomatoes, wine and garlic (minced); bring to a simmer.
- Return beef and accumulated juices to Dutch oven.
- Cover and bake 2 1/2 hours, stirring once halfway through cooking time, until beef is very tender.
- One serving is about 3/4-1 cup.

Easy Beef Brisket

Ingredients

- 1/2 lb Beef Brisket (Whole, Lean Only)
- 1/4 tsp Salt
- 1/4 tsp Paprika
- 1/8 tsp Black Pepper
- 1/2 tbsp Sugar Free Apricot Preserves

Directions

- Heat oven to 475F.
- Season brisket with salt, paprika and pepper.
- Place brisket fat side down in a Dutch oven.
- Scatter onions and carrots around the beef.
- Cook 15 minutes.
- Turn brisket fat side up and add 1/2 cup water.
- Cover tightly.
- Reduce oven temperature to 375°F.
- Cook 3 to 4 hours, until brisket is fork tender.
- Heat broiler.
- Remove brisket from Dutch oven and place on a broiler pan.

- Spread jam over brisket.
- Broil 6 from heat source 5 minutes, until jam is lightly browned in spots.
- While brisket is broiling, remove onions and carrots from cooking juices.
- Cover brisket with foil and allow to rest 15 minutes before serving.
- Remove surface fat with a spoon and serve with de-greased cooking juices.

Beef Salad with Edamame

Ingredients

- 1 medium (4-1/8" long) Scallions or Spring Onion
- 1/4 tsp Garlic
- 1/2 tbsp Tamari Soybean Sauce
- 1/4 tbsp Sodium and Sugar Free Rice Vinegar
- 1/4 tsp Toasted Sesame Oil
- 1/8 tsp Sucralose Based Sweetener (Sugar Substitute)
- 4 1/4 ozs Beef Top Sirloin (Trimmed to 1/8" Fat, Choice Grade)
- 1/8 tsp Curry Powder
- 1/16 tsp Ginger (Ground)
- 1/2 tbsp Canola Vegetable Oil
- 3/4 cup Spring Mix Salad
- 1/4 medium (approx 2-3/4" long, 2-1/2" dia) Red Sweet Pepper
- 2 ozs Water Chestnuts
- 1/2 cup Shelled Edamame

Directions

- Mix green onions, garlic, soy sauce, rice wine vinegar, sesame oil and sugar substitute in a small bowl.
- Pour half into a resealable plastic bag; add steak and marinate overnight in the refrigerator.
- To remaining soy sauce mixture, add curry powder and ground ginger.
- Heat canola oil in a large skillet over high heat until very hot.
- Drain beef and discard marinade; quickly stir-fry beef 2 to 3 minutes in hot oil.
- Transfer to a large mixing bowl.
- Add salad greens, bell pepper, water chestnuts, edamame and reserved soy dressing.
- Toss to coat.

Low Carb Lobster Salad

Ingredients

- 1/2 lb Northern Lobster
- 1 cup shredded Chinese Cabbage (Bok-Choy, Pak-Choi)
- 1/4 small Sweet Red Pepper
- 2 medium (4-1/8" long)s Scallions or Spring Onions
- 1/2 tbsp Dried Whole Sesame Seeds
- 1 tbsp Sodium and Sugar Free Rice Vinegar
- 1 tbsp Tamari Soybean Sauce
- 1/2 tbsp Canola Vegetable Oil
- 1/2 tsp Sesame Oil
- 1/2 tsp Ginger

Directions

- For the salad: In a large serving bowl, combine lobster, cabbage, bell pepper, scallions and sesame seeds.

- For the dressing: In a small bowl, whisk the rice vinegar, Tamari soy sauce, ginger and sesame and canola oils together.
- Pour dressing over salad and toss gently to coat.
- Season with fresh ground black pepper and salt.

Chinese Tuna Kebabs

Ingredients

- 2/3 tbsp Tamari Soybean Sauce
- 2/3 tbsp Sodium and Sugar Free Rice Vinegar
- 1/8 tbsp Toasted Sesame Oil
- 1/8 tbsp Ginger
- 1/2 tsp Garlic
- 1/4 tsp Sugar Substitute
- 4 oz boneless Tuna
- 1/2 large Scallions or Spring Onion
- 1/8 large Red Sweet Pepper
- 1/8 lb Eggplant

Directions

- Heat grill to high.
- Combine soy sauce, rice wine, sesame oil, ginger, garlic and sugar substitute in a large bowl.
- Add tuna, scallions and red pepper and toss to coat.
- Marinate for 15 minutes in the refrigerator.

- Remove tuna, scallions and red pepper from marinade and set aside.
- Toss eggplant in marinade and let sit for 3 minutes.
- Remove eggplant and set aside with other ingredients.
- Discard marinade.
- Thread skewers, alternating 3 pieces of tuna, 2 pieces of scallions, 2 pieces of red pepper and 3 pieces of eggplant on each.
- Eggplant should be skewered through both skin sides of the rounds.
- Grill for 3 4 minutes per side tuna will be rare in the center.

Asparagus & Leek Soup

Ingredients

- 1/2 tbsp Unsalted Butter Stick
- 1/4 leek Leeks
- 1/4 lb Asparagus
- 1/4 tsp Garlic
- 1/4 14.5 oz can Chicken Broth
- 1/8 cup Heavy Cream

Directions

- Melt butter in a large pot over medium-high heat.
- Add leeks and sauté for 3 minutes.
- Add asparagus and cook 1 minute more.
- Add garlic and sauté for 30 more seconds.
- Add broth to pot and bring to a boil.
- Lower heat, cover and simmer 8 to 10 minutes, until asparagus is tender.
- Mix in cream, salt and pepper.

- Blend soup in a food processor or blender until smooth.
- Return to pot to heat through before serving.
- Season with salt and freshly ground black pepper to taste.

Asparagus & Tarragon Soup

Ingredients

- 1/8 tbsp Extra Virgin Olive Oil
- 1/2 14.5 oz can Chicken Broth
- 1/4 lb Asparagus
- 1/2 stalk medium Celery
- 1/16 tsp Salt
- 1/16 tsp Black Pepper
- 1/8 small Onion
- 1/16 tbsp leaf Tarragon
- 1/8 cup Heavy Cream

Directions

- Heat oil in a large pot over medium-high heat.
- Add white onion and cook 5 minutes, until softened but not browned.
- Add broth, asparagus, celery, salt, pepper and half of the tarragon to the pot. Bring to a boil.
- Lower heat, cover and simmer 20 minutes, until asparagus is very tender.
- In a blender, puré soup in batches until smooth.

- Return to pot.
- Add cream and remaining tarragon and heat soup through over medium heat.
- Season with salt and freshly ground black pepper

Sausage Pizza With Bell Peppers and Onions

Ingredients

- 1/4 tsp Baking Powder
- 1/8 individual packet Sugar Substitute
- 1/8 cup Tap Water
- 1/2 tbsp Extra Virgin Olive Oil
- 1/16 cup Tomato Sauce
- 1/8 small Red Onion
- 1/16 medium Red Sweet Pepper
- 1/16 tsp Salt
- 1/16 medium Green Sweet Pepper
- 1/8 cup shredded Whole Milk Mozzarella Cheese
- 3/4 serving All Purpose Low-Carb Baking Mix
- 1/8 link (5" long) Italian Sausage

Directions

- Preheat oven to 425°F.
- Blend together baking mix, baking powder, salt and sugar substitute in a large mixing bowl.
- Add water and oil.

- Using a wooden spoon or a spatula, combine into a dough.
- Using a spatula, remove the dough from the bowl and place on a clean surface lightly coated with olive oil spray.
- Coat rolling pin with oil spray and roll the dough out to fit the pizza pan or stone.
- Or use your hands to pat the dough into shape.
- Bake the crust for 10 minutes and remove from oven.
- Spread tomato sauce evenly over the pizza.
- Sprinkle with mozzarella and top with sausage rounds, green and red bell pepper slices and onions.
- Sprinkle with salt and pepper to taste.
- Return to the oven and continue baking for 10-15 minutes.
- Cut into 8 slices.

Low Carb Yorkshire Pudding

Ingredients

- 1/16 cup Whole Grain Soy Flour
- 1/4 oz Vital Wheat Gluten
- 1/3 large Egg (Whole)
- 1/8 cup Whole Milk
- 1/8 tsp Salt
- 1/16 cup Canola Vegetable Oil
- 1/8 tsp Baking Powder (Straight Phosphate, Double Acting

Directions

- Preheat oven to 450° F.
- Whisk together soy flour, gluten, eggs, milk and salt.
- Pour drippings or oil into an 8-inch square baking dish, and place on center rack in oven for 5 minutes, until drippings or oil is smoking hot. Then add batter and bake 15 minutes.
- Lower temperature to 350° F and bake for 15 to 20 minutes more, until lightly browned.

- Serve piping hot.

Printed in Great Britain
by Amazon